Veterinarian's Guide to Maximizing Biopsy Results

Veterinarian's Guide to Maximizing Biopsy Results

F. Yvonne Schulman
DVM, Diplomate ACVP

WILEY Blackwell

This edition first published 2016 © 2016 John Wiley & Sons, Inc.

Editorial offices: 1606 Golden Aspen Drive, Suites 103 and 104, Ames, Iowa 50010, USA
        The Atrium, Southern Gate, Chichester, West Sussex, PO19 8SQ, UK
        9600 Garsington Road, Oxford, OX4 2DQ, UK

For details of our global editorial offices, for customer services and for information about how to apply for permission to reuse the copyright material in this book please see our website at www.wiley.com/wiley-blackwell.

Library of Congress Cataloging-in-Publication Data applied for.
ISBN: 9781119226260

A catalogue record for this book is available from the British Library.

Wiley also publishes its books in a variety of electronic formats. Some content that appears in print may not be available in electronic books.

Set in 9.5/13pt, MeridienLTStd by SPi Global, Chennai, India.
Printed and bound in Malaysia by Vivar Printing Sdn Bhd

1   2016

Contents

Preface: Why maximizing your biopsy results is important

A biopsy is the collection of tissue to be analyzed by the pathologist. It is often the gold standard of diagnosis. Ideally, from the pathologist's perspective, all lesions would be biopsied so that treatment could be based on a confirmed diagnosis. However, as with most decisions, the decision to perform a biopsy should be based on a cost-benefit analysis. The costs include time, biopsy procedure fee, histology fee, pet discomfort, possible infection or spread of disease, and owner inconvenience. The potential benefits are an accurate diagnosis and prognostic information to guide future treatment, decrease patient suffering, and avoid the cost of treating an assumed incorrect condition. There are many steps in the biopsy process that can be optimized to ensure minimizing the cost and maximizing the benefit. This manual is designed to help clinicians submit cost-effective biopsies by providing suggestions for each step of the biopsy submission, separate organ specific biopsy considerations, a step-by-step biopsy submission checklist, and a list of general biopsy dos and don'ts. It is hoped that this manual provides enough detail to be helpful, but not so much that the useful information is obscured, and that it will be consulted often prior to biopsy collection.

Acknowledgments

I gratefully acknowledge Drs. Thomas Lipscomb and Frances Moore for helpful comments on the manuscript, Dr. Anne Kincaid for helping to collect case material, Ms. Ingrid Style for her advice on the drawings, Mr. Lance Schuette and Ms. Pam Schmidt for scanning slides, Marshfield Laboratory histology technicians for some of the gross photos, Dr. Michelle Fleetwood for help with the literature review, and Julie, Mary, and Charles Lipscomb for their encouragement.

Steps of a Successful Biopsy Submission

1 Collection

Each step of the biopsy submission process is important and contributes to the accuracy of the diagnosis, but the collection step is critical. While submission form information can be added to or revised at a later date and the correlation between the histologic and clinical assessments can be reassessed as new information is provided, the quality of the biopsy specimen is irrevocably determined by the collection method. One cannot make up for improper collection or fixation with a longer clinical history.

i Site

When presented with a single, small lesion, the site selection is straightforward (Figure 1), but when lesions are disseminated or the lesion is very large (Figure 2), site selection can make the difference between collection of diagnostic and non-diagnostic samples. When multiple lesions are present, take a sample from more than one as more than one disease may be present. In cases of widespread skin disease, sample several sites to get a range of the lesions. Areas of necrosis, ulceration, and secondary infection should be avoided as they often obscure the primary lesion (Figure 3). Be sure to biopsy any intact vesicles or pustules. For lesions that are too large to excise, multiple biopsies, including all grossly different appearing areas, are recommended in an attempt to submit fully representative specimens.

ii Size

While the type of biopsy specimen collected (such as needle, punch, incisional or excisional biopsies (Figures 4–7), endoscopic or full-thickness specimens) depends on many factors, that is, size of the lesion, type and accessibility of

Veterinarian's Guide to Maximizing Biopsy Results, First Edition. F. Yvonne Schulman.
© 2016 John Wiley & Sons, Ltd. Published 2016 by John Wiley & Sons, Ltd.

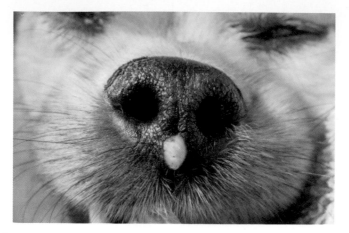

Figure 1 Solitary mass, viral papilloma, on the nose of a terrier. A single excisional biopsy was diagnostic and curative. (Reproduced by permission of Bass Lake Pet Hospital, New Hope, MN 55428).

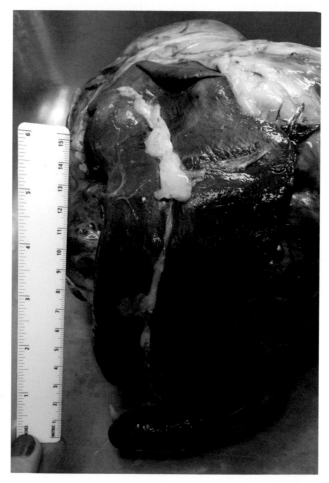

Figure 2 Spleen (in the foreground) with a large mass attached to the far side that requires sampling of all grossly different appearing areas to fully evaluate the lesion.

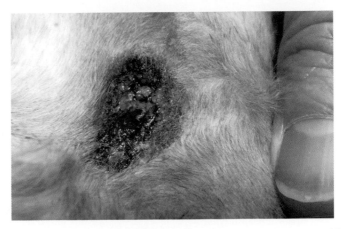

Figure 3 Ulcerated skin lesion (feline squamous cell carcinoma in situ [Bowen's-like disease] in this case). Excisional biopsy or sampling the periphery of the lesion is more likely to be diagnostic than a biopsy of the central ulcerated area. (Reproduced by permission of Whitewater Veterinary Hospital, Whitewater, WI 53190).

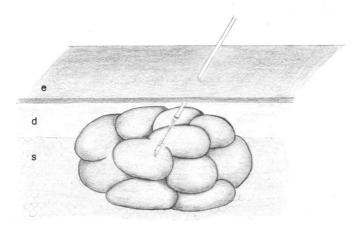

Figure 4 Drawing of a needle biopsy of a skin mass sampling a small proportion of the lesion. e = epidermis, d = dermis, and s = subcutis.

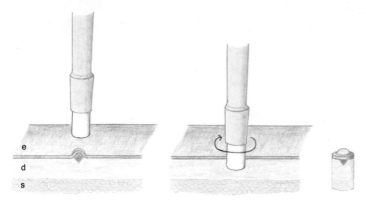

Figure 5 Drawing of the punch biopsy procedure. The punch biopsy instrument is placed over the lesion, rotated in one direction while avoiding excessive pressure and results in a cylindrical specimen. e = epidermis, d = dermis, and s = subcutis.

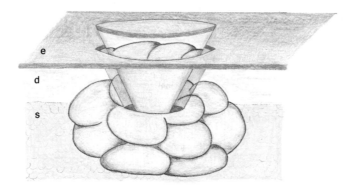

Figure 6 Drawing of an incisional biopsy of a skin mass sampling more than a needle biopsy, but less than an excisional biopsy. e = epidermis, d = dermis, and s = subcutis.

tissue, health of the patient, and so on, the certainty of submitting a representative specimen and, therefore, getting an accurate diagnosis, is proportional to the percentage of the lesion biopsied (Figure 8). In other words, the larger the biopsy sample, the more likely it is to be fully representative and diagnostic. When clinically reasonable, excisional biopsies are recommended. Not only are excisional biopsies fully representative of the lesion, but they can also be curative.

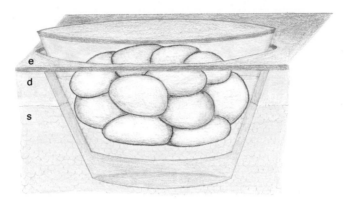

Figure 7 Drawing of an excisional biopsy of a skin lesion with removal of the entire lesion, providing (i) a fully representative specimen, (ii) the best chance at reaching an accurate diagnosis, and (iii) possibly a cure. e = epidermis, d = dermis, and s = subcutis.

Whenever possible, include some of the apparently normal surrounding tissue. The interface between the lesion and unaffected tissue often provides important information for interpreting the lesion, such as maturation of reactive tissue, well-circumscribed margin of benign neoplasms, or invasive growth of malignant tumors (Figures 9–12).

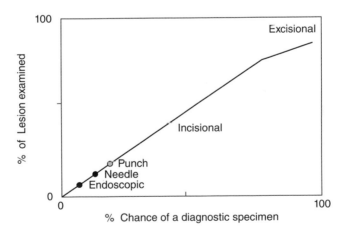

Figure 8 Graph of size of biopsy vs. likelihood of submitting a diagnostic specimen. The greater the percentage of the lesion submitted, the more likely the specimen will be fully representative and diagnostic (modified graph from Stromberg, P.C. (2009) *The principles and practice of veterinary surgical pathology*. CL Davis Foundation Workshop. ACVP Annual Meeting. Monterey, CA. Adapted with permission from Dr. Paul Stromberg.).

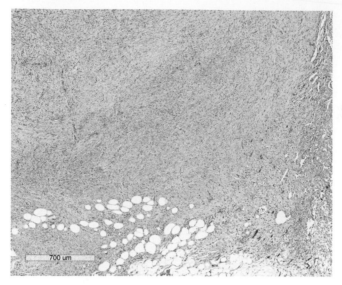

Figure 9 Photomicrograph of the peripheral maturation of granulation tissue and blending of the lesion with the adjacent connective tissue, a feature that helps distinguish this reactive lesion from a spindle cell neoplasm.

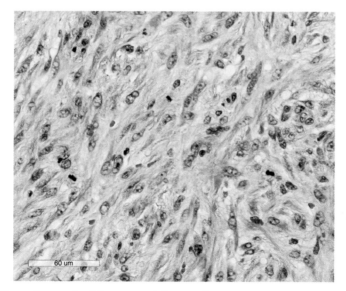

Figure 10 Photomicrograph of the center of the granulation tissue in Figure 9. These mitotically active, immature spindle cells can easily be misinterpreted as a malignant spindle cell neoplasm if the margins of the lesion cannot be evaluated.

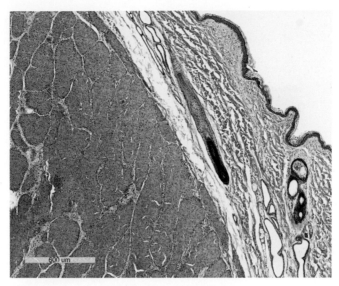

Figure 11 Photomicrograph of a portion of the smooth margin of a benign tumor (a circumanal [also called perianal or hepatoid] adenoma in this case). The tumor (left) and adjacent haired skin (right) are included in the specimen.

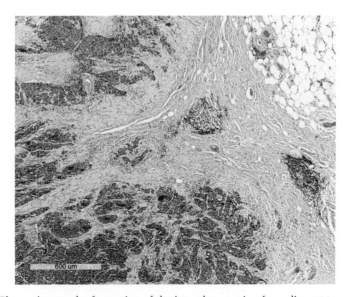

Figure 12 Photomicrograph of a portion of the irregular margin of a malignant tumor. The tumor (left) is invading the adjacent fibroadipose tissue (right). Neoplastic tissue is surrounded by a fibroblastic reaction (desmoplasia).

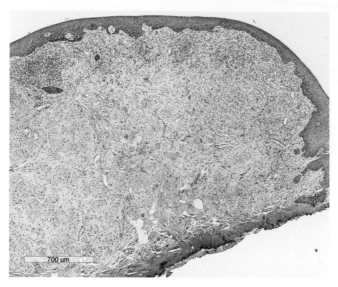

Figure 13 Photomicrograph of an oral mucosal biopsy with coagulation of the tissue margin (bottom right), consistent with electrocautery or laser-induced artifact and characterized by amorphous tissue and loss of detail. As the specimen is relatively large and only the margin was affected, the specimen is diagnostic (a sparsely pigmented oral melanocytic neoplasm in this case).

Be careful to avoid artifacts. Small specimens are especially susceptible to tissue coagulation and squeeze artifact. Electrocautery and lasers coagulate tissue, forming an amorphous residuum. In larger specimens, only the tissue margins are affected (Figure 13), leaving an area of viable, potentially diagnostic tissue, but in smaller specimens, the entire sample can be rendered non-diagnostic (Figures 14 and 15).

To avoid squeeze artifact, use sharp cutting blades and handle tissues gently, avoiding or minimizing the use of forceps. A new biopsy punch is indicated for each patient to ensure a sharp blade. Lymphoid cells rupture easily (Figures 16 and 17). If lymphoma is suspected, be particularly gentle during collection and submission of the specimens. Forceps squeeze/crush tissue, causing tissue distortion and rupturing cells (Figures 18–22). Tiny tissue fragments wrapped in gauze can be difficult to find and may be distorted during retrieval.

Some recommend the use of tissue cassettes with cassette foam sponges (Figures 23 and 24) for submission of small specimens, but when fresh tissue is placed in cassettes with cassette sponges, the sponges impale the tissue, forming triangular spaces, which distorts the tissue, rupturing cells and hampering histologic evaluation (Figures 25–28). If the specimens are so small that they will be lost through the small slits or pores in the tissue cassettes, they are usually of limited diagnostic value, and if possible, larger specimens should be obtained. When cassettes with cassette sponges are to be used, the tissue specimens should be fixed prior to placement in the cassettes, or in cases of

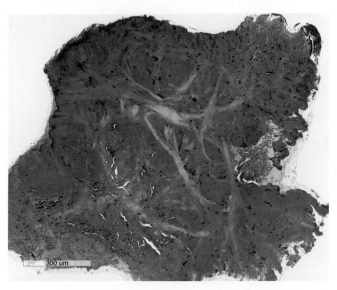

Figure 14 Photomicrograph of a diffusely coagulated specimen with loss of detail (consistent with electrocautery or laser-induced artifact), resulting in unrecognizable tissue.

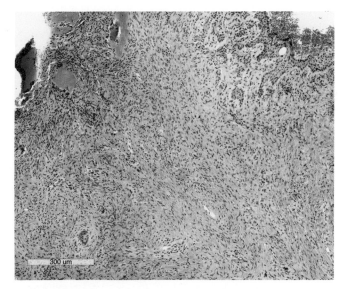

Figure 15 Photomicrograph of uncoagulated tissue from the same lesion as in Figure 14. This specimen reveals what the tissue looked like before coagulation and is diagnostic of a fibromatous epulis.

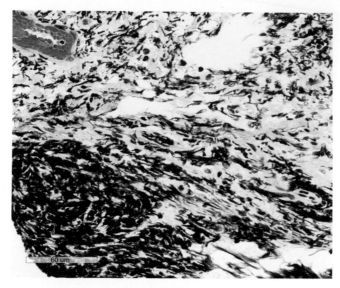

Figure 16 Photomicrograph of lymphoid tissue with squeeze artifact induced at the time of biopsy collection. The cells have ruptured, resulting in streaming chromatin (blue streaks) and precluding cell identification.

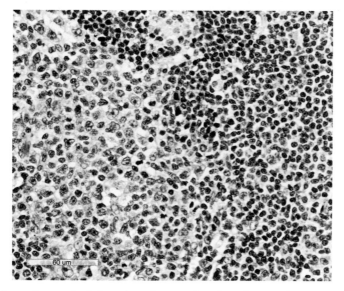

Figure 17 Photomicrograph of tissue from the same lymph node as in Figure 16 without squeeze artifact. The cells of the lymphoid follicle (left) and paracortical area (right) are intact and recognizable.

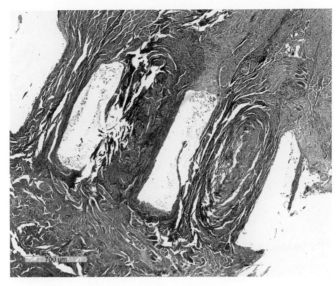

Figure 18 Photomicrograph of tissue distorted by a clamp, resulting in rectangular spaces and greatly hampering tissue identification and histologic evaluation.

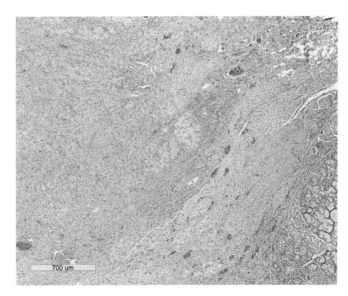

Figure 19 Photomicrograph of the same tissue as in Figure 18 without the clamp-induced artifact, revealing reactive fibroplasia involving fibrovascular tissue and skeletal muscle. Salivary gland tissue is present in the lower right.

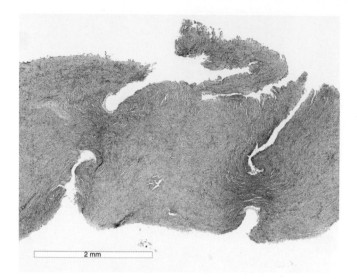

Figure 20 Photomicrograph of tissue distorted by forceps, resulting in two areas of sharp tissue constriction.

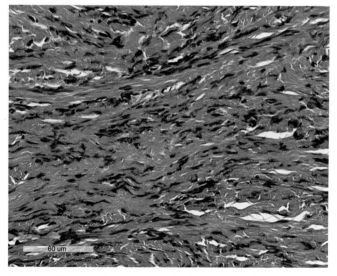

Figure 21 Higher-magnification photomicrograph of a constricted area of the tissue in Figure 20, demonstrating the squeeze artifact caused by the forceps. The cells have ruptured, resulting in streaming chromatin (blue streaks) and precluding cell identification.

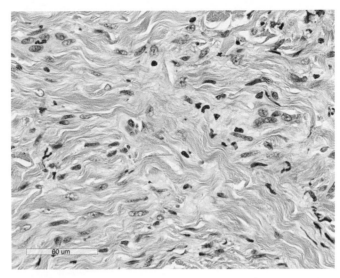

Figure 22 Higher-magnification photomicrograph of an unconstricted area of the tissue in Figure 20, demonstrating what the tissue looks like without the artifact induced by the forceps and revealing plump fibroblast separated by collagen.

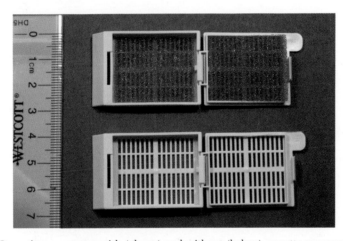

Figure 23 Open tissue cassettes with (above) and without (below) cassette sponges.

small endoscopic or needle biopsy specimens, wetting the sponges with formalin before placing the tissue in the cassette can result in good-quality samples.

iii Number

The number of biopsies taken depends on the number and distribution of the lesions, as well as the size of biopsy, with the aim of submitting representative tissue. An excisional biopsy of a single lesion requires only a single specimen; however, if punch or core biopsies are taken of a large lesion, more than one

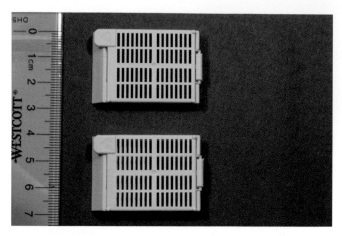

Figure 24 Closed tissue cassettes.

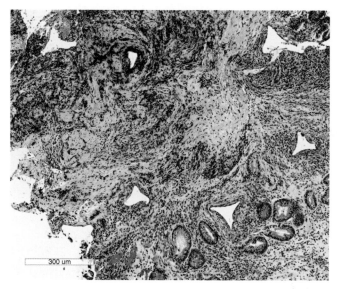

Figure 25 Photomicrograph of rectal mucosa submitted in a tissue cassette with cassette sponges. The sponges have impaled the tissue producing triangular clear spaces, distorting the tissue, rupturing cells, and greatly hampering histologic evaluation.

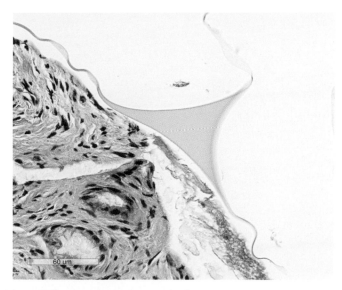

Figure 26 High-magnification photomicrograph of cassette sponge material, which demonstrates the triangular portion that causes the characteristic artifact seen in Figures 25 and 27.

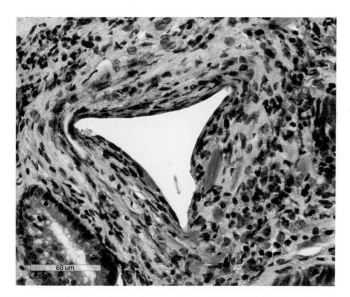

Figure 27 Higher-magnification photomicrograph of a characteristic triangular clear space in Figure 25 caused by submission of unfixed tissue in cassettes with dry cassette sponges. The tissue is distorted, hampering histologic evaluation of the tissue architecture and cell types present.

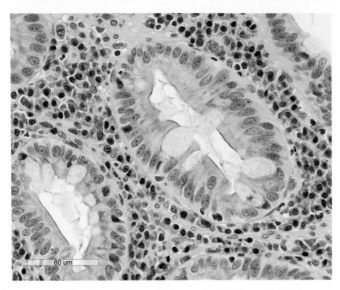

Figure 28 Photomicrograph of rectal tissue similar to that in Figure 27 without cassette sponge-induced artifact. The tissue architecture is intact, the epithelium can be properly assessed, and plasma cells and occasional lymphocytes are evident in the lamina propria.

biopsy should be taken to increase the percentage of the lesion sampled and the probability of obtaining fully representative specimens. In cases of widespread disease or multiple lesions, multiple biopsies are recommended. Lesions may be at different stages, some of which are more diagnostic than others, and all lesions may not be the result of the same disease.

Do not submit multiple specimens and ask the pathologist to choose the ones to examine. The clinician, who has the whole patient to examine, is in a better position to choose representative specimens for histologic evaluation than the pathologist or technician examining formalin-fixed tissues. Most diagnostic laboratories will process each tissue that is submitted.

iv Fixation

In general, for routine histologic evaluation, tissues should be placed in neutral buffered 10% formalin immediately after collection to prevent desiccation, autolysis (Figures 29–32) and bacterial overgrowth. Use at least 10:1 formalin to tissue volume. To avoid shipping large amounts of formalin, specimens can be shipped post-fixation in just enough formalin to keep them moist. Proper fixation requires at least 24 hours (different tissues have different rates of formalin fixation). If the specimen will be subjected to freezing temperatures, add one part 95% ethyl alcohol to nine parts formalin in order to prevent freeze artifact. Freezing causes ice crystals to form in the tissue, resulting in tissue clefts and distortion (Figures 33 and 34) and hampering histologic evaluation.

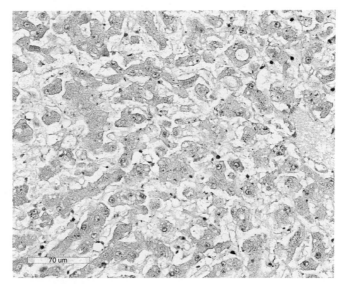

Figure 29 Photomicrograph of autolytic liver. There is loss of cellular detail with altered staining quality, cell shrinkage, and indistinct chromatin.

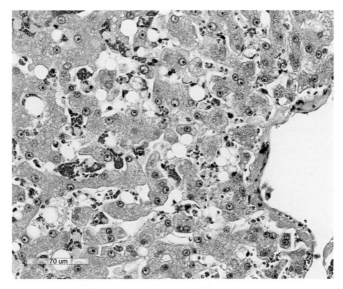

Figure 30 Photomicrograph of liver tissue that was fixed promptly and lacks significant autolytic changes. The cells are larger and exhibit more nuclear and cytoplasmic details than the autolytic tissue in Figure 29.

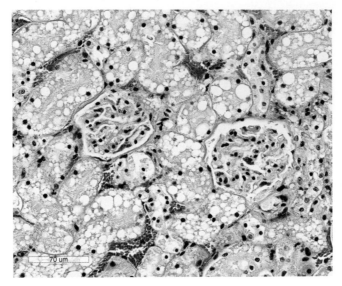

Figure 31 Photomicrograph of autolytic kidney. There is loss of cellular detail with altered staining quality, cell shrinkage, and small dark nuclei that can be misinterpreted as necrosis.

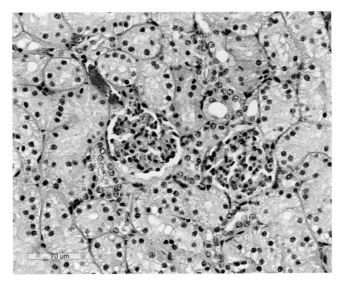

Figure 32 Photomicrograph of kidney that was fixed promptly and lacks significant autolytic changes. The cells are larger and exhibit more nuclear and cytoplasmic details than the autolytic tissue in Figure 31.

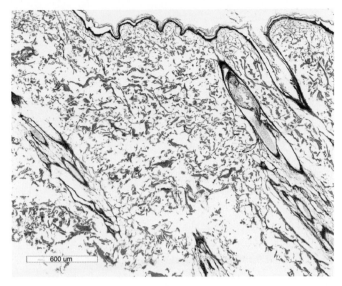

Figure 33 Photomicrograph of haired skin with freeze artifact. There are numerous tissue clefts (clear spaces) distorting the dermis.

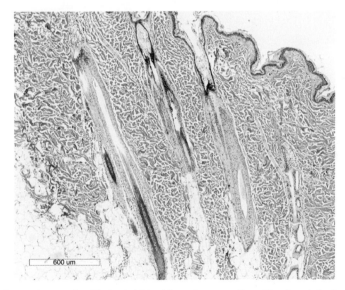

Figure 34 Photomicrograph of haired skin without freeze artifact. The dermis lacks the relatively large tissue clefts seen in the tissue that was frozen in Figure 33.

Specimens should be less than 1 cm thick to allow adequate penetration of the tissue by the formalin. The following techniques can be used to allow for adequate tissue fixation of larger specimens:

a. Incomplete serial sectioning ("breadloafing") (Figure 35) - Make incomplete (to maintain tissue orientation), parallel cuts, preferably less than 1 cm apart.

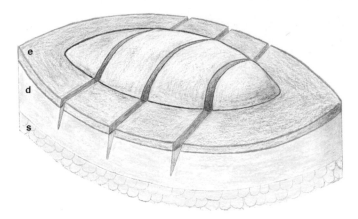

Figure 35 Drawing of an excisional biopsy specimen of a cutaneous mass that has incomplete, parallel incisions (has been "breadloafed") to allow for rapid fixation of the tissue while maintaining tissue orientation and integrity of the surgical margin. e = epidermis, d = dermis, and s = subcutis.

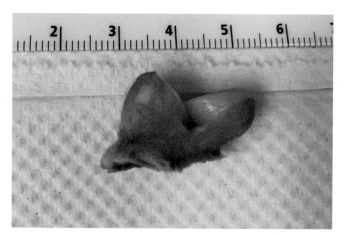

Figure 36 Side view of an excisional biopsy specimen of a skin mass that has been incompletely incised from the surface to allow for rapid fixation of the tissue while maintaining tissue orientation and integrity of the surgical margin.

Inking margins of interest should be done prior to breadloafing to prevent ink from adhering to non-surgical margins. When incompletely incising skin specimens, make the incision(s) through the skin surface and not the subcutis to maintain the integrity of the surgical margin (Figure 36).

b. Splitting the sample - Ink the surgical margins with India ink or commercially available tissue marking dyes prior to cutting the specimen to allow for orientation and reassembly of the specimen during histologic processing and assessment of completeness of excision.

c. Subsampling - Take representative samples of large specimens from at least three different sites to include all grossly different appearing areas.

If special testing is a consideration, additional tissue can be cultured, frozen (for toxicology, metal analysis or PCR), snap frozen (for molecular diagnostics), or placed in glutaraldehyde (for electron microscopy).

v   Labeling and packaging

Submit tissue in leak proof and shatterproof, wide-mouthed containers labeled with the names of animal, owner, and veterinarian/clinic (Figures 37–39). If submitting more than one tissue, be sure to include the tissue source on the label. Glass jars can break and should not be used. The label should be affixed to the container and not the lid. Make sure the widest part of the specimen fits through the narrowest part of the container. After fixation, the specimen becomes rigid and cannot squeeze through narrow openings that it could before it was fixed.

Ideally, each specimen should be submitted in its own container. If submitting multiple specimens in one container, each specimen should be clearly differentiated by different numbers of sutures, different suture colors, different colored inks, or truly unique morphologic features. The site of endoscopic or needle biopsy samples can be indicated by submitting them in labeled cassettes; however, as indicated above, cassette sponges can impale fresh tissue, causing significant tissue artifacts. If there is a risk of the tissue escaping from the tissue cassette, cassette sponges can be used (after they have been wet with formalin or the specimens have been fixed) or Cellsafe™ biopsy capsules can be used instead of cassette sponges, but tissues this small are often of limited diagnostic use. Specimens submitted on cardboard or tongue depressors frequently become

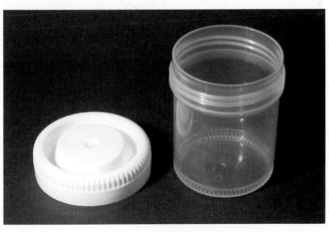

Figure 37 An example of a leak proof and shatterproof, wide-mouthed container for biopsy specimens.

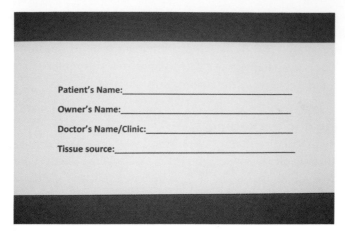

Figure 38 An example of a label template that includes prompts for the names of the animal, owner, and doctor/clinic, as well as the tissue source.

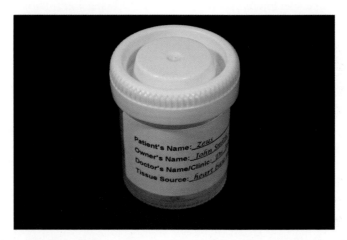

Figure 39 An example of a biopsy container with a label including the appropriate information attached to the container and not the lid.

detached, and transporting specimens this way does not provide a reliable way of labeling tissues.

Different lengths, numbers or colors of sutures, or different colors of ink can also be used to indicate orientation of the specimen (Figure 40) and different margins of interest (Figures 41, 42).

Federal shipping regulations must be observed when transporting biological specimens (U.S. Department of Transportation 2007; American Veterinary Medical Association 2015). Biopsy specimens require triple packaging with (i) a primary watertight container, (ii) watertight secondary packaging with sufficient absorbent material to absorb the entire liquid contents, and (iii) sturdy, ridged walled outer packaging. All individuals involved in the packaging and shipping

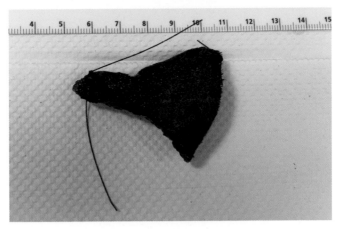

Figure 40 A skin biopsy specimen with a long suture and a short suture indicating different margins. The long suture marks the cranial margin and the short suture the dorsal margin.

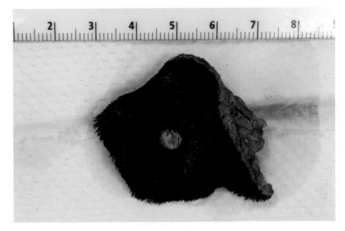

Figure 41 The superficial aspect of an excisional skin biopsy specimen marked with different colored inks to indicate different margins.

of infectious substances must have proper training, and packages must be appropriately labeled.

2 Submission form

Clinicians are busy professionals, but it is very important to take the time to provide the pathologist with the basic background information with which to interpret the histologic findings. The pathologist usually does not have access to the patient and depends on the clinician to provide the medical facts of the case. The biopsy captures a tiny percentage of the patient and often a small

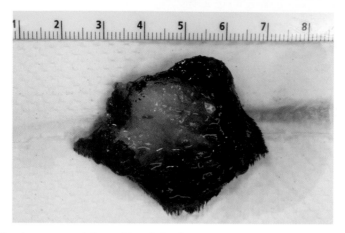

Figure 42 The deep aspect of the excisional skin biopsy specimen in Figure 41 marked with different colored inks to indicate different margins. The red ink marks the cranial margin, green ventral, black caudal, and blue dorsal.

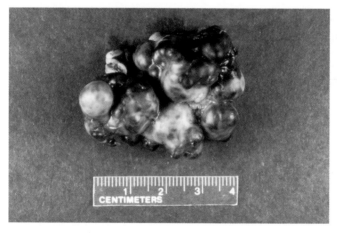

Figure 43 A botryoid (cluster of grapes-shaped) mass from the base of the heart of a dog that was diagnosed histologically as hemangiosarcoma.

percentage of the tissue/mass being evaluated. Missing information reduces the specificity and/or certainty of the pathologist's diagnosis.

i Signalment and clinical history

Species, breed, sex (intact or neutered), and age are important. "Bird" is not a signalment. The clinical history should be succinct and include pertinent clinical signs, any previous treatment, response to treatment, and whether others in the environment are affected. Do not waste time with extraneous details, but make sure you explain why you are taking the biopsy.

ii   Lesion description

Reporting that "a lesion" was biopsied does not impart any useful information. Bearing in mind that the pathologist usually cannot examine the patient, describe the lesion as if to a person who cannot see, touch or smell. The following list of attributes should be addressed in your description:

a. Number, location, and distribution – Please be specific regarding location. When given "abdomen" as the location, the pathologist doesn't know if the lesion is from the skin, subcutis, mammary gland, skeletal muscle, peritoneum, lymph node, or any of the abdominal viscera.

b. Size – Objective size is always best, but comparison to sizes of common items, such as dime-sized, is better than no size reference. Avoid relative terms, such as "large" and "small."

c. Color

d. Shape – ovoid, spherical, conical, flat, nodular, discoid, botryoid (Figure 43), and so on.

e. Consistency – soft, firm, hard, resilient, friable, viscous, mucoid, gritty, homogeneous, and so on.

f. Other – discrete or ill-defined, fixed or movable, ulcerated or not, malodorous and so on.

When possible, photographs of the lesion(s) in situ can be a very helpful addition to the biopsy submission material.

iii   Differential diagnosis and specific questions

When provided with your differential diagnosis, the pathologist can specifically address whether or not the histologic findings support the conditions on the list. Asking specific questions on the submission form is the most efficient way to get answers to questions the pathologist might not anticipate and address in his/her report.

3   Clinicopathologic correlation

In most cases, the pathologist has no direct contact with the patient and depends on the information you provide on the submission form. Your pathologist will attempt to correlate that information with the histologic findings to reach a diagnosis, differential diagnosis, and/or offer suggestions for additional steps/testing to reach a more specific diagnosis. The histologic diagnosis should be reviewed in light of the clinical signs, physical exam, other laboratory tests, and response to treatment. If the pathologist's conclusions do not correlate well with your clinical assessment, please contact the pathologist to discuss the discrepancy. Additional biopsies should be considered if the lesion appears to recur, if the condition does not respond appropriately to the recommended treatment, or to track response to treatment.

Organ System Specific Guidelines

1 Skin

Skin lesions are easily visualized, readily accessible, and relatively easily biopsied. Skin biopsies do not require expensive equipment and generally do not require complicated procedures. Skin biopsy sites in most veterinary patients typically heal well.

Skin lesions can be focal, multifocal or widespread, and cutaneous or subcutaneous. If there are no clinical contraindications, focal lesions that are small enough for excisional biopsy should be excised. If excisional biopsy is not feasible, securing an incisional biopsy of an area as large as possible or multiple punch biopsies is indicated. Skin punch biopsies of subcutaneous lesions generally provide little if any of the lesional tissue and are not recommended (Figure 1). If lesions are multifocal or widespread, multiple biopsies are recommended.

Clinicians should remember that biopsies of non-mass skin lesions frequently do not yield a specific diagnosis, but rather a morphologic diagnosis that can be used in combination with the clinical information to stratify the differential diagnosis, redirect the clinical workup, and guide therapy.

Special considerations for skin punch biopsies:

i. If possible, biopsy before treatment. Treatment can alter the histologic lesion, rendering it non-diagnostic. If corticosteroids have been given and if not contraindicated by the patient's condition, corticosteroids should be withdrawn for at least 2 weeks prior to biopsy.

ii. If widespread disease, take multiple biopsies demonstrating the range of lesion stages and appearances, including active and older lesions. If present, biopsy pustules, vesicles, macules, papules, and crusts.

iii. Avoid areas that are diffusely or deeply ulcerated, secondarily infected, or scarred. The primary lesion will be masked.

iv. Do not scrub the skin surface. Scrubbing can remove crusts/parasites and rupture pustules/vesicles that may be critical in reaching a diagnosis. Skin punch biopsy procedures are clean but not sterile procedures, and may be contraindicated if the patient is immune compromised or predisposed to septicemia.

Veterinarian's Guide to Maximizing Biopsy Results, First Edition. F. Yvonne Schulman.
© 2016 John Wiley & Sons, Ltd. Published 2016 by John Wiley & Sons, Ltd.

   v. If using local anesthesia, be sure to inject the lidocaine into the subcutis and not the dermis to avoid causing an artifact that can histologically mimic edema.

  vi. Use a new punch biopsy instrument for each patient. Dull blades can cause tissue compression and squeeze artifact. Use the cutting action of the tool by rotating in one direction and avoid excessive pressure. Six-millimeter punches are more informative than 4-mm punches (Figures 2 and 3). Four-millimeter punches should be reserved for the nasal planum, footpads, and very small lesions.

 vii. Place what you want the pathologist to evaluate in the center of the punch. During tissue processing, punch biopsies are usually bisected and the center of the specimen ends up on the slide for examination (Figure 4).

viii. Handle the specimen gently. Do not squeeze the tissue with forceps (Figures 5–7).

  ix. Immediately gently blot and float the specimen in formalin. Small skin punch biopsy specimens can fit in labeled cassettes without cassette sponges to identify different sites of collection or stages of the disease. Do not squeeze fresh tissue in a cassette with a dry cassette sponge, which will impale the tissue, producing triangular clear spaces in the specimen and hampering histologic evaluation.

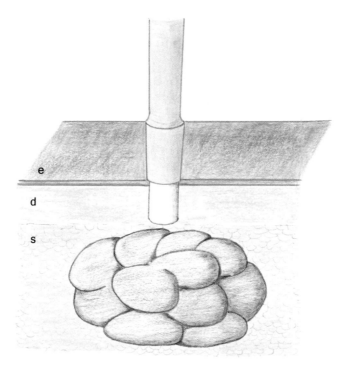

Figure 1 Drawing of a punch biopsy that cannot adequately sample a subcutaneous mass. e = epidermis, d = dermis, and s = subcutis.

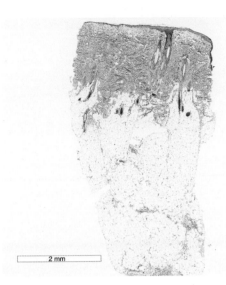

2 mm

Figure 2 Photomicrograph of a good-quality 4-mm skin punch biopsy specimen. The amount of tissue and number of adnexal units is significantly smaller than in a 6-mm (Figure 3) or 8-mm punch biopsy specimen, reducing the likelihood of a fully representative sample and decreasing the chance of reaching a specific diagnosis. This specimen has non-specific histologic changes.

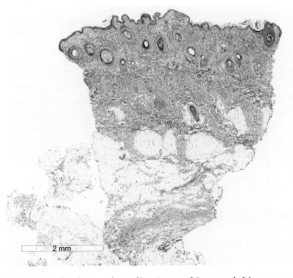

2 mm

Figure 3 Photomicrograph of a good-quality 6-mm skin punch biopsy specimen that includes more tissue and adnexal units than a 4-mm (Figure 2) punch biopsy specimen, increasing the amount of tissue examined and the likelihood of reaching a specific diagnosis, in this case demodicosis.

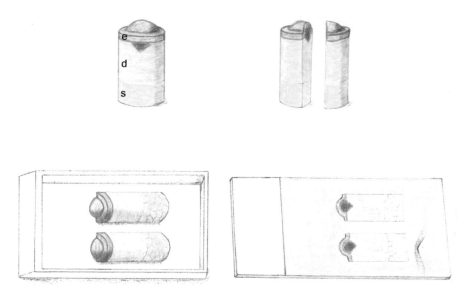

Figure 4 Drawing of how a skin punch biopsy is processed for histology. The punch is bisected and the bisected sections laid flat in a tissue cassette. This results in the center of the specimen being represented on the glass slide. e = epidermis, d = dermis, and s = subcutis.

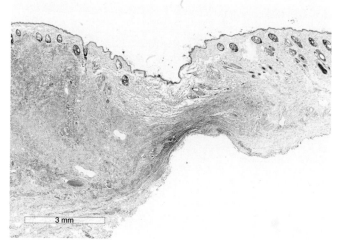

Figure 5 Photomicrograph of a skin biopsy specimen with a focal narrowing caused by forceps. The tissue in the affected area is squeezed/crushed, resulting in significant tissue distortion.

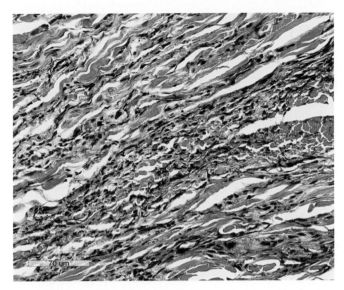

Figure 6 Higher-magnification photomicrograph of the area squeezed by the forceps in Figure 5. The cells have ruptured, resulting in streaming chromatin (blue streaks) and precluding cell identification.

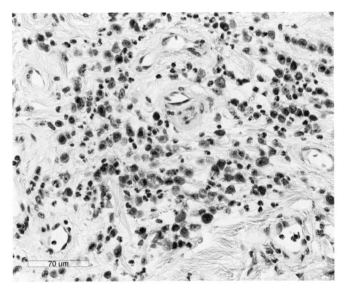

Figure 7 Higher-magnification photomicrograph of the area not affected by the squeeze artifact in Figure 5. The unruptured cells are recognizable as well-differentiated neoplastic mast cells and eosinophils.

2   Mammary

Mammary gland tumors are common in female dogs, cats, and rats. They are also not uncommon in guinea pigs, both male and female. These tumors are readily apparent and accessible.

Histologic differentiation between benign and malignant mammary tumors depends largely on examination of the tumor margins for the presence or absence of invasive growth (Figures 8 and 9). Therefore, cytology, needle biopsies, and incisional biopsies are often of limited diagnostic use. Excisional biopsy to include surrounding normal tissue is generally the best way to diagnose and treat mammary tumors.

Female dogs frequently develop multiple different mammary tumors (Sorenmo *et al.* 2009), and submission of one mammary tumor will not tell you what the other mammary tumors are. In addition, mammary tumors can undergo malignant transformation over time (Sorenmo *et al.* 2009). Prompt excisional biopsy of all mammary tumors is usually recommended.

The one exception to the recommendation for excisional biopsy of all mammary tumors is canine inflammatory mammary carcinoma due to the associated grave prognosis and short survival time (Susaneck *et al.* 1983). This tumor presents as a rapidly spreading area of erythema and heat with nodules, plaques, or increased firmness to the tissue. Histologically, it is usually an adenocarcinoma with extensive lymphatic invasion, areas of infiltrating, individualized anaplastic cells with a fibroblastic reaction, and mild inflammation (Figure 10). A punch or incisional biopsy can be used to differentiate inflammatory mammary carcinoma from mastitis.

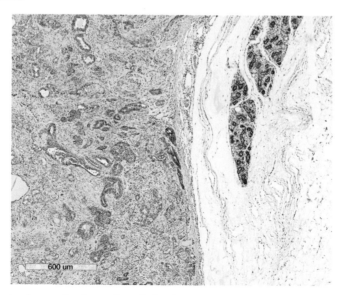

Figure 8 Photomicrograph of a portion of a benign mammary gland tumor (complex adenoma on the left) with a smooth margin and adjacent mammary gland tissue (right).

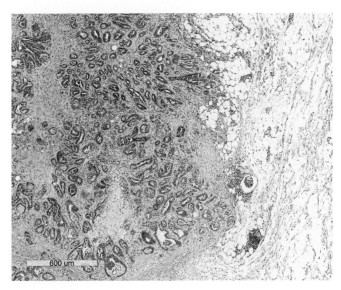

Figure 9 Photomicrograph of a portion of a malignant mammary gland tumor (simple adenocarcinoma on the left) with an invasive, irregular margin surrounded by a fibroblastic reaction and adjacent fibroadipose tissue (right).

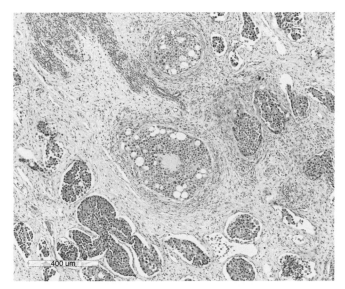

Figure 10 Photomicrograph of canine inflammatory mammary carcinoma. Anaplastic cells infiltrate tissue (center) and fill and distend lymphatics (aggregates of blue cells surrounded by clear spaces around the periphery). Mammary tissue is present (upper left).

3 Oral

Lesions in the oral cavity are less visible and accessible than those of the skin and mammary gland tissue and obtaining appropriate biopsy specimens of these lesions can require surgical expertise. Because of the difficulty of collecting biopsies from the oral cavity, submitted samples are often small, superficial, and/or fragmented, making histologic interpretation difficult. In addition to submitting the largest specimens possible given the clinical situation, the following considerations may help maximize the information to be gleaned from the samples that you collect:

  i. When submitting oral lesions, be sure to report whether or not there is bone involvement. If the bone is involved, describe the radiographic findings and/or submit the radiographs. If osteolysis is present, submit samples from the osteolytic area(s).

 ii. Be aware that biopsies of inflamed gingiva are frequently unrewarding. The inflammation is usually stereotypical, composed of many plasma cells and neutrophils with fewer lymphocytes, and not specific as to cause (Figure 11).

iii. Submission of teeth is rarely diagnostic. Submit the tissue around the tooth.

 iv. If taking a biopsy of an ulcerated lesion, there is bound to be inflammation and granulation tissue that can mask any underlying disease. Increasing the depth of the biopsy and/or sampling adjacent non-ulcerated tissue may increase the likelihood of identifying any underlying lesions.

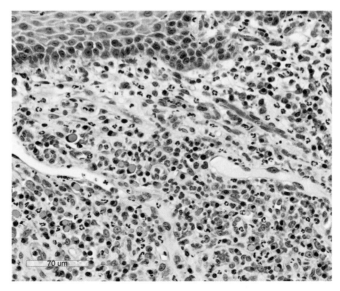

Figure 11 Photomicrograph of feline gingivitis. Many plasma cells with fewer neutrophils and scattered Mott cells (immunoglobulin-distended plasma cells) are typically seen and are not specific as to cause.

v. Electrocautery or lasers are often used for oral mucosal biopsies to help control bleeding, but it must be remembered that these techniques coagulate tissue and can render small specimens non-diagnostic. If using these techniques to remove a small lesion, use a scalpel to remove it and then cauterize the base or take wider margins to ensure a diagnostic specimen.

In cases of partial mandibulectomy/maxillectomy, there is frequently a previous histologic diagnosis that has led to the surgery and the primary purpose of submission is to determine completeness of excision. It is helpful to indicate which margins the surgeon is most concerned with in that regard. Colored ink, sutures, or a clear verbal description can be used to indicate to the histology technician and/or pathologist which areas to evaluate.

4 Gastrointestinal tract

The gastrointestinal tract is more difficult to access and biopsy than skin or mammary gland tissue. It requires specialized instrumentation and techniques, increasing the cost. Endoscopy allows for direct, minimally invasive visualization and biopsy of the gastrointestinal mucosa, but an inherent limitation of endoscopic biopsies is their small size. Therefore, it is especially important to consider the following recommendations to provide the best specimens for the pathologist to interpret and maximize your results:

i. Endoscopic biopsies sample a tiny percentage of the mucosa (Figure 12). Take multiple (6–10) biopsies of each site.

ii. Larger and deeper biopsies allow for better orientation of the specimen and evaluation of more tissue, including both superficial and deep mucosa (Figures 13 and 14). Using pinch forceps with larger cups and applying pressure to the mucosa with the biopsy instrument at the time of biopsy yields larger and deeper specimens. Suction is another method to enhance the size and depth of the mucosal samples.

iii. Handle tissue carefully to minimize squeeze artifact. Fenestrated forceps are reported to cause less squeeze artifact than non-fenestrated instruments (Golden 1993). Once the specimen is collected, gently tease it from the forceps with a needle. The specimens can then be placed on a formalin-soaked cassette sponge with the deep surface against the sponge for orientation and immediately placed in formalin (Willard *et al.* 2001) or directly placed in formalin. Do not put fresh specimens in cassettes with dry cassette sponges. Dry sponges impale fresh tissue, causing significant artifacts.

iv. Samples from different sites should be submitted in different containers and labeled appropriately.

v. Remember that endoscopic biopsies of the gastrointestinal tract only sample the mucosa plus or minus the muscularis mucosa. If the lesion is deeper than that, it will be missed with this technique (Figure 15). Full-thickness

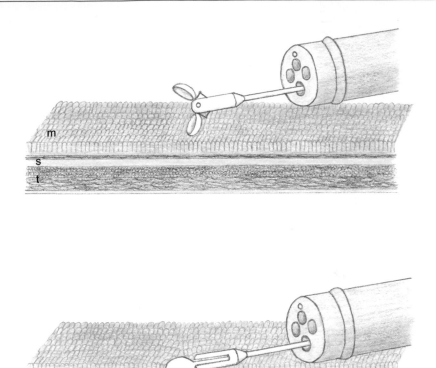

Figure 12 Drawing of an endoscopic biopsy procedure. The endoscopic forceps collect a very small percentage of mucosa plus or minus submucosa. m = mucosa, s = submucosa, t = tunica muscularis.

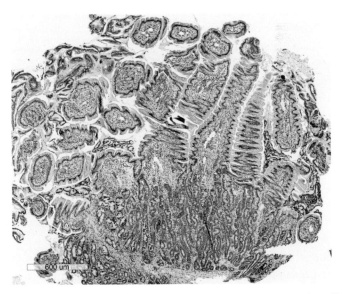

Figure 13 Photomicrograph of a good-quality endoscopic biopsy specimen of small intestine. The sample includes superficial (villi) and deep (crypts) mucosa with no significant squeeze artifact.

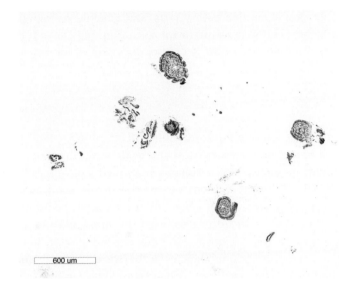

Figure 14 Photomicrograph of poor-quality endoscopic biopsy specimen of small intestine. Only villi were collected. These specimens can be lost during tissue processing, provide excessively small amounts of tissue for evaluation and preclude examination of the deep mucosa.

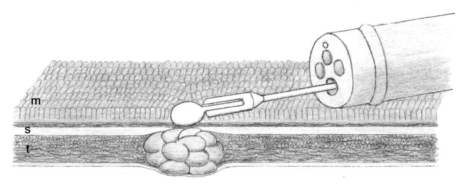

Figure 15 Drawing of how endoscopic biopsy specimens cannot adequately sample a mural lesion. m = mucosa, s = submucosa, t = tunica muscularis.

biopsies allow for evaluation of all layers of the tract and more consistent proper orientation of the specimens during processing, ensuring more accurate assessment of superficial and deep mucosa.

   vi. In cases of feline chronic small bowel disease, endoscopic biopsy specimens may not be adequate for differentiating between inflammatory bowel disease and low-grade, small-cell lymphoma, and full-thickness biopsies are recommended (Evans *et al.* 2006; Norsworthy *et al.* 2015).

   vii. Correlate the clinical signs with the endoscopic observations and histologic findings. The histologic findings must be interpreted in light of the clinical history, physical exam, laboratory tests, and possibly radiographic studies. Animals lacking endoscopic and histologic lesions may have functional disease, such as motility disorders, secretory disorders, or enzyme deficiencies.

5   Liver

Liver biopsies provide important information in diagnosing a patient with hepatic disease, as well as determining prognosis and evaluating response to treatment. Because the liver produces most coagulation factors, liver disease can lead to bleeding tendencies. Some liver diseases cause disseminated intravascular coagulation (DIC) and consumption of coagulation factors. In addition, prolonged obstruction of bile flow can lead to decreased intestinal absorption of vitamin K1, an important cofactor of clotting. Therefore, patients with hepatic disease should be assessed for bleeding tendencies. If there is clinical evidence of bleeding, the risk of biopsy-associated hemorrhage should be carefully considered. If liver biopsy is still considered critical to the diagnosis, blood products should be on hand to deal with potential hemorrhage.

Ideally, the structure of the liver, bile duct, and portal vein should be evaluated via ultrasound, laparoscopy, or surgical exploratory prior to biopsy. The information gleaned from this examination, including size of liver, focal, multifocal or diffuse nature of the lesion, presence or absence of abdominal fluid, and so on, should be included in the submission form to aid the pathologist in interpretation of the biopsy. A clinical history of "Liver" conveys no useful information and greatly limits histologic interpretation, especially in the case of needle biopsies.

When considering which sites to biopsy, be aware that liver margins, being furthest from the main blood supply, are predisposed to fibrosis. This fibrosis can mask underlying disease, or in the face of limited clinical information, be over-interpreted as more widespread hepatic fibrosis. Sometimes grossly normal appearing areas are actually abnormal and vice versa, so sample both the grossly abnormal and normal areas. Large focal lesions should be sampled at the periphery to avoid possible necrotic tumor centers and to evaluate the interaction of the lesion with the adjacent normal tissue.

Liver biopsies usually evaluate only a small percentage of the liver and may not be fully representative. Types of liver biopsies include needle, punch, wedge, lumpectomy, and lobectomy. The smaller the specimen, the less tissue architecture is available for evaluation. While it depends on the size of the patient and their liver, one good needle biopsy is estimated to represent 1/50,000 of the liver in humans (Gellar 1994). In one study, needle biopsy and wedge biopsy diagnoses of the same liver lobe did not agree in about 50% of cases (Cole *et al.* 2002). Many needle biopsies do not yield complete hepatic lobules and have few portal triads and/or centrilobular veins. Needle biopsies are not recommended if congenital vascular disorders of the liver are suspected, as histologic diagnosis of these conditions requires examination of multiple hepatic lobules and portal triads. Biopsies of small nodular livers are usually not indicated, as those livers are end-stage livers for which the cause is generally no longer evident and the prognosis is poor.

When liver needle biopsies are taken, remember:

i. The larger the needle diameter, the more architecture will be seen. 14 G needle biopsies can be obtained from most dogs and 16 G from small dogs and cats.

ii. Always take multiple biopsies.

iii. If the lesion is widespread or diffuse throughout the liver, take biopsies from different lobes.

iv. Handle tissue specimens carefully to avoid squeeze artifact and fragmentation of the specimens.

v. Submission in tissue cassettes can help prevent fragmentation of the specimens in transit. If using cassette sponges, presoak them with formalin to avoid artifact.

vi. If sampling mass lesions, be sure to indicate the number and size of the lesions.

6 Pancreas

Pancreatic biopsy is generally considered the gold standard for the diagnosis of pancreatitis. It can also be used for diagnostic and therapeutic purposes in cases of pancreatic neoplasia. While postoperative complications can occur following pancreatic surgical biopsy, good surgical techniques, including gentle tissue handling, can minimize the risk (Pratschke *et al.* 2015). Unlike in human medicine where endoscopic and ultrasound-guided biopsy/aspiration is generally used when sampling the pancreas, in veterinary medicine, this technique has not proved reliable (Cordner *et al.* 2010) and most pancreatic biopsies are collected during exploratory abdominal surgery.

As pancreatitis can result in small, discrete lesions with no preferential sites, a single biopsy sample may not identify pancreatic disease. If only one biopsy is to be taken in cases of a grossly normal pancreas or diffuse disease, the distal right limb is the recommended sample site because of the distance from the duct system, vascular supply and ready surgical access (Cornell & Fischer 2003). Wedge biopsy with a scalpel blade, suture fracture, or blunt dissection and ligation technique can be used (Cornell & Fischer 2003). Crushing the pancreas with hemostats can release pancreatic enzymes, increasing the risk of postoperative pancreatitis, and should be avoided.

Pancreatic enzymes predispose pancreatic tissue to autolysis. As with almost all biopsy specimens, pancreatic biopsies should immediately be placed in formalin.

It should also be remembered that an absence of histologic lesions in the biopsy specimen, especially if only one sample is submitted, does not necessarily mean the patient does not have pancreatic disease. The biopsy results must be interpreted in conjunction with the clinical findings and other diagnostic tests.

7 Spleen

Biopsy of the spleen is usually prompted by splenomegaly or splenic masses. Splenic masses often contain extensive areas of congestion, hemorrhage, necrosis, inflammation, and/or fibrosis that can mask underlying disease, making adequate sampling paramount (Figures 16–19).

Needle biopsies of the spleen are often non-diagnostic. Partial or complete splenectomy is diagnostic and can be therapeutic. If a splenic mass is too large to submit in toto, submission of at least three <10-mm-thick sections, including all grossly different-appearing areas, is recommended. Include a section of the mass with adjacent normal tissue. The periphery of the mass usually has more viable tissue. If multiple masses are present, biopsy more than one, as different lesions can be present in the same spleen.

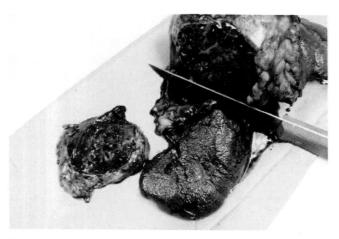

Figure 16 A splenic mass with areas of congestion, necrosis, and hemorrhage. Thin slices (less than 1 cm) including all grossly different-appearing areas allow for proper fixation and adequate sampling to identify the lesion (hemangiosarcoma in this case). (Reproduced by permission of Dr. Steven Ekholm, Walker Animal Hospital, Walker, MN 56484).

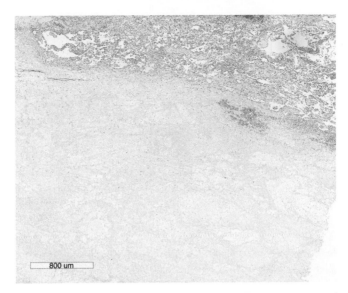

Figure 17 Photomicrograph of a splenic hemangiosarcoma with extensive necrosis (bottom two thirds). The viable neoplastic tissue (upper one third) was at the periphery of the mass. Sampling only the center of the tumor would be non-diagnostic.

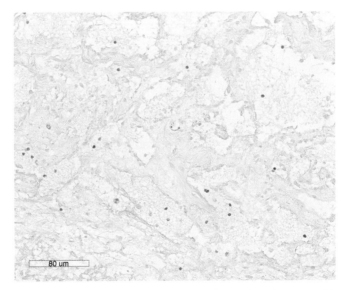

Figure 18 Photomicrograph of the center of the tumor depicted in Figure 17. This necrotic tissue is non-diagnostic.

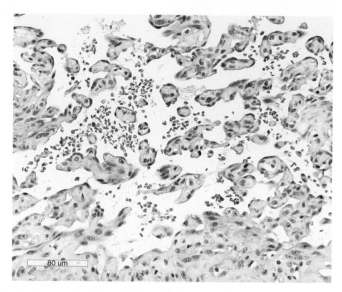

Figure 19 Photomicrograph of the periphery of the tumor depicted in Figure 17. This viable area of the tumor is diagnostic of hemangiosarcoma.

8 Lymph nodes

Lymph nodes are typically biopsied because of lymph node enlargement or to check for spread of a neoplasm. Submission of the entire lymph node allows proper evaluation of the lymph node architecture, aiding in recognition of tissue effacement by lymphoid neoplasms and identification of lesions that may only affect a portion of the lymph node. Many lymph nodes that contain neoplasia or areas of infection also have areas of reactive lymphoid hyperplasia, thus partial sampling of a lymph node can result in an incomplete diagnosis (Figure 20). As mentioned before, lymphoid cells are especially prone to cell rupture. Submission of the whole lymph node, in addition to gentle handling, can help minimize squeeze artifact.

In cases of lymphadenopathy affecting multiple lymph nodes, biopsies of more than one lymph node are recommended. This increases the percentage of affected tissue evaluated, increases the likelihood of an accurate diagnosis, and helps address the possibility of more than one disease process.

Occasionally, subjectively enlarged lymph nodes that drain a site of primary interest, such as a mesenteric lymph node in a case of enteritis or a popliteal lymph node associated with a digital mass, are submitted instead of the primary lesion. The lymph node is frequently expanded by reactive lymphoid hyperplasia

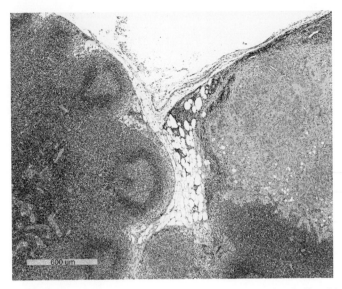

Figure 20 Photomicrograph of a lymph node that is focally infiltrated and effaced by metastatic neoplasia (mammary adenocarcinoma) on the right. The rest of the lymph node is expanded by reactive lymphoid hyperplasia. A partial biopsy of the lymph node could easily miss the neoplastic tissue and lead to a diagnosis of only lymphoid hyperplasia.

and plasmacytosis that are not specific as to cause and provide no useful information about the primary lesion. The primary tissue of interest should always be biopsied.

9   Bone

Bone biopsies are usually performed because of a mass lesion and/or osteolysis. Bone lesions are often presumptively diagnosed via radiographs and clinical findings, but biopsy, or less commonly, cytology is used to reach a definitive diagnosis. Bone biopsy specimens should always be accompanied by a description of the radiographic lesion and/or the radiographs. Another reason for bone biopsy is to evaluate bone marrow in cases of abnormal CBC results.

Core biopsies, limb-sparing procedures, or amputation can be used to obtain bone specimens. Core biopsies sample a limited amount of tissue, and when taken by those inexperienced in bone core biopsy technique, are often non-diagnostic due to insufficient sample size or non-representative specimens (Figures 21 and 22). When taking a core biopsy of a bone lesion, take multiple biopsies and sample the osteolytic area(s), as well as the junction between the

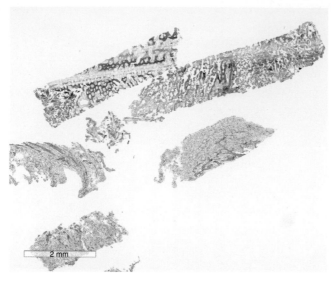

Figure 21 Photomicrograph of good-quality bone core biopsy specimens, allowing for the identification of a neoplasm (osteosarcoma in this case) filling the intertrabecular spaces.

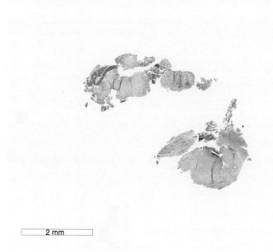

Figure 22 Photomicrograph of poor-quality bone core biopsy specimens. The samples are primarily composed of periosteal fibrovascular tissue with a tiny amount of bone (brighter pink areas) and are non-diagnostic.

osteolytic and normal bone, to increase the likelihood of collecting a diagnostic specimen.

Amputation specimens are generally too large to fix properly if left undissected in formalin. They should be kept cool with ice packs and delivered promptly to the pathology laboratory for processing. As the time period between amputation and tissue fixation increases, the degree of autolysis increases and the diagnostic quality of the specimen decreases (Figures 23 and 24). If the amputation specimen includes a soft tissue lesion, representative samples of the affected soft tissue should be placed in formalin as soon as possible and submitted with the rest of the specimen.

Decalcification is required for histologic processing of most bone specimens. This process takes time, and a longer turnaround time should be expected.

When the purpose of the biopsy is to evaluate bone marrow, the tissue specimen should always be accompanied by a concurrent bone marrow aspirate and complete blood count (CBC). While the biopsy can evaluate overall cellularity of the bone marrow, marrow architecture, and the presence of absence of necrosis and myelofibrosis, the aspirate allows for better evaluation of individual cell morphology, aiding in identification of cell lineages and dysplasias, and in the assessment of myeloid to erythroid and maturation ratios. The biopsy and aspirate findings must be interpreted in light of the CBC results and clinical history.

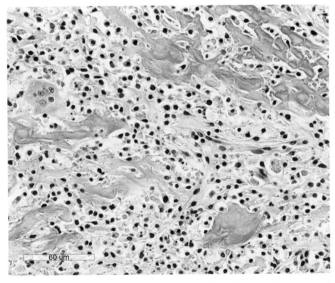

Figure 23 Photomicrograph of autolytic osteosarcoma. The cells are shrunken with significant loss of nuclear detail compared to osteosarcoma without autolysis (Figure 24).

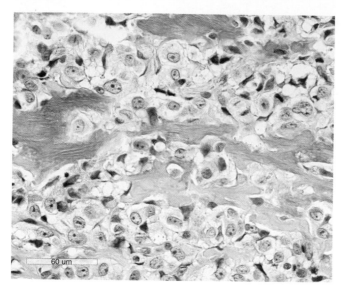

Figure 24 Photomicrograph of osteosarcoma without autolysis. Neoplastic cells are not shrunken and nuclear details are clear in comparison to autolytic osteosarcoma (Figure 23).

10   Digits

Biopsies of digits are usually performed in cases of chronically swollen and painful digits, mass lesions, or claw abnormalities. Clinical presentations of benign neoplasms, malignant neoplasms, and inflammatory lesions of the digits can be similar; histopathology is generally required to differentiate between them. Lumpectomies in this location can be associated with difficulty in closing the surgical defect. Smaller biopsies are often not fully representative of the lesion. Amputation is commonly used to both diagnose and treat digital lesions in the dog and cat.

Complete histologic evaluation of amputated digits requires extra time for decalcification of the bones, so a delay in the results should be anticipated.

In the vast majority of cases of multiple, brittle, deformed, and/or sloughing claws in a dog, the histologic findings are those of lupoid onychitis (onychodystrophy), which is believed to represent a stereotypic inflammatory reaction pattern affecting the nailbed in a variety of conditions, such as food hypersensitivity, drug reaction, nutritional deficiencies, and so on. The histologic lesions of lupoid onychitis involve the nailbed epithelium and can be patchy. Therefore, amputation of the distal phalanx is often required to adequately sample the lesion. Submission of the claw(s) with little or no nailbed epithelium generally does not provide a diagnostic specimen; however, as almost all cases of progressive deformity and loss of claws on multiple paws in the absence of systemic signs or other lesions have histologic features consistent with lupoid onychitis, the presumptive diagnosis can be made from the clinical presentation.

Bacteria and aggregates of degenerate neutrophils are commonly seen in the stratum corneum of the claw in biopsy specimens, but bacterial infections of the claw are usually secondary to some other condition. Submission of only the claw will not help identify the underlying disease. Fungal infections involving only the claw are rare.

11 Eyes

Eyes can be enucleated (removal of the globe) or eviscerated (removal of the contents of the globe). Common causes for these procedures include glaucoma, ocular neoplasia, trauma and endophthalmitis. In veterinary medicine, most eyes are enucleated. If a tumor is present, evisceration is not recommended as the likelihood of incomplete excision is increased with this procedure. Other ocular specimens include biopsies of the cornea, conjunctiva, and third eyelid.

If removing an eye for histopathology, remove it as quickly as possible while maximizing the patient's safety and comfort. All adnexa except the third eyelid (which is helpful for orientation of the specimen during tissue processing) not requiring histologic evaluation should be trimmed off of the globe; the intact eye should immediately be placed in fixative. Do not incise or inject the eye with fixative, as this can distort ocular structures and cause tissue artifacts. Different pathologists/laboratories prefer different fixatives for eyes. Formalin, Bouin's solution, or Davidson's solution can be used. Contact your laboratory to find out their preference.

12 Urinary

i Kidney

Renal biopsies can be helpful in reaching a diagnosis and providing information regarding the severity, chronicity, activity, and potential reversibility of renal disease. However, renal biopsies are not without risks and these biopsies should only be undertaken when the results are likely to alter patient management and after careful consideration of any contraindications.

Indications for renal biopsy include protein-losing nephropathies and acute renal failure. Biopsies are not indicated in cases of end stage renal disease associated with small kidneys. At this stage, the cause is generally not evident, the disease is usually irreversible and progressive, and the biopsy results will not change the treatment, that is, supportive care.

The most common complication of renal biopsy is hemorrhage (Valden *et al*. 2005). Hydronephrosis, renal infarction, fibrosis, vascular changes, infection, and death are also possible. To avoid complications, renal biopsy should not be performed on animals that have uncorrectable coagulopathies, severe

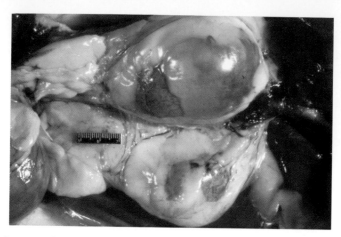

Figure 25   A large renal cyst (upper kidney) is a contraindication for renal needle biopsies.

anemia, hydronephrosis, hypertension, large or multiple renal cysts (Figure 25), perirenal abscess or extensive pyelonephritis (Valden 2005; Lees *et al.* 2011), or on dogs that weigh less than 5 kg (Valden *et al.* 2005).

Ultrasound is useful in assessing the size, shape, and internal features of the kidney, and should be performed prior to renal biopsy to help rule out some of the contraindications listed above. The ultrasound findings should be conveyed to the pathologist on the biopsy submission form to aid in interpretation of the histologic findings. Ultrasound is also recommended for percutaneous biopsies of the kidney to guide correct placement of the needle (Valden 2005).

Only cortical tissue should be collected. The risk of serious hemorrhage and infarction increases if the corticomedullary junction is crossed; arcuate arteries located at the corticomedullary junction can be damaged by biopsy needles (Figures 26–29). Additionally, evaluation of glomeruli, which reside in the cortex, is often the primary purpose of the biopsy procedure.

At least two cortical cores at least 10 mm long or three cores less than 10 mm long should be submitted (Lees *et al.* 2011). Sharp 16- or 18-gauge needles can be used for collection, but 16-gauge needles provide more tissue for evaluation, and are, therefore, more informative. Prior to submission for histopathology, needle biopsy specimens of kidney can be assessed with a dissecting microscope, ocular loop, or handheld lens, and a good light source to insure cortical tissue was sampled. During this process, the specimens should be kept moist with physiologic saline and handled with great care to avoid producing squeeze artifact.

Alternatively, a wedge biopsy of cortex can be submitted. Wedge biopsies provide more tissue for evaluation and are less subject to fragmentation and squeeze artifact.

Light microscopy may be all that is needed for diagnosis, but complete evaluation of glomeruli often requires electron and immunofluorescent microscopy. If these additional examinations are anticipated, the collected renal cortical tissue

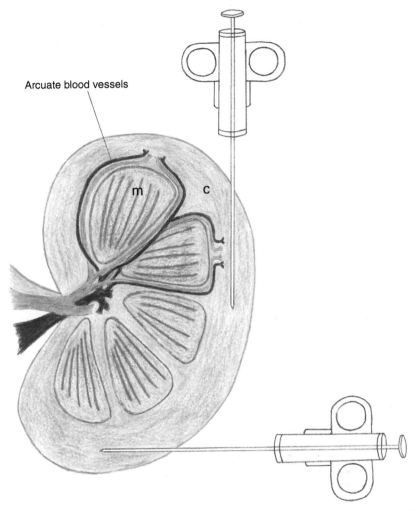

Figure 26 Drawing of correct approaches for needle biopsies of the kidney, sampling only the cortex and avoiding the arcuate blood vessels. c = cortex and m = medulla.

should be subdivided. The bulk of the specimen should be placed in formalin for light microscopy. Specimen(s) <2 mm in greatest dimension should be put in glutaraldehyde for electron microscopy, and another piece should be frozen or placed in Michael's fixative for immunofluorescence.

ii Bladder and urethra

The best indication to biopsy the urinary bladder or urethra is a mass lesion. Biopsies of the urinary bladder of cats that have clinical signs of cystitis are generally unrewarding, revealing slightly thickened urothelium with little if any inflammation, consistent with chronic mucosal irritation.

Arcuate blood vessels

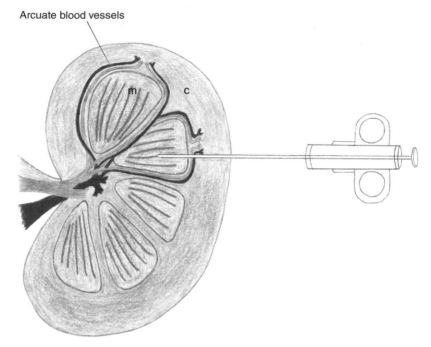

Figure 27 Drawing of the incorrect approach for needle biopsies of the kidney, crossing the corticomedullary junction, possibly puncturing the arcuate blood vessels and causing hemorrhage. c = cortex and m = medulla.

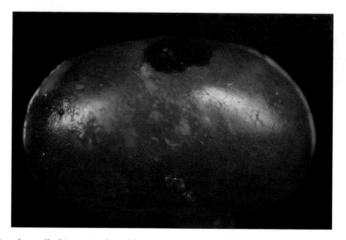

Figure 28 Focal needle biopsy-induced hemorrhage in the kidney of a tree kangaroo.

While catheter and cystoscopy biopsies of the bladder and urethra can yield diagnostic results and are less invasive and expensive than surgical biopsies, the small size of the samples collected with a catheter increases the possibility of a non-diagnostic specimen or a less specific diagnosis. Not only are excisional biopsies fully representative of the lesion, but they can also be curative.

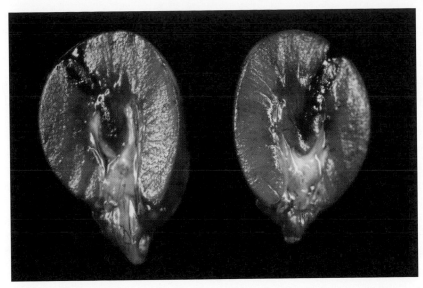

Figure 29 Linear hemorrhagic tracts in the same kidney depicted in Figure 28. The hemorrhage was caused by a misdirected needle biopsy that crossed the corticomedullary junction.

13   Respiratory

i   Nasal

Nasal biopsies are most commonly performed in cases of chronic nasal discharge and/or nasal masses. Clinical history, physical exam, and blood work should be used to rule out systemic or extranasal causes of the discharge, such as coagulopathies, vasculitis, hypertension, and pneumonia. Imaging studies should always be performed prior to rhinoscopy and/or biopsy because they can be used to help guide the rhinoscopic and biopsy procedures and the procedures can cause hemorrhage that may interfere with interpretation of the images.

Whenever possible, computed tomography (CT) is the imaging study of choice for the nasal cavity. It is superior to conventional radiography in detecting changes in the nasal cavity, determining the extent of the lesion and differentiating neoplastic disease from rhinitis. Unlike rhinoscopy that can only access a limited area of the nasal cavity, CT can evaluate the entire nasal cavity and adjacent structures. CT is preferred over magnetic resonance imaging (MRI) because of the higher cost of MRI and better evaluation of bony structures by CT.

Different techniques for nasal biopsies include blind intranostril biopsy collection using forceps or bone curette, otoscopic illuminator-assisted biopsy of rostral lesions, rhinoscopy-guided biopsy, CT image-based biopsy, sinus trephination, open-rhinotomy, and aggressive nasal flushing/nasal hydropulsion. Blind biopsies of mass lesions may be larger than biopsies obtained during rhinoscopy, which are limited by the size of the instrument that can be introduced alongside the rhinoscope, and are frequently diagnostic in cases of nasal mass lesions (Harris *et al.* 2014). Nasal hydropulsion is minimally invasive and can obtain relatively large specimens, providing immediate clinical relief and a high success rate for definitive diagnosis of suspected intranasal tumors (Ashbaugh *et al.* 2011).

Nasal biopsies collected with forceps are small, and gentle tissue handling to avoid squeeze artifact is essential to maximize the amount of histologically interpretable tissue. If nasal lymphoma is suspected, extra care is warranted as lymphoid cells are easily ruptured. For submission of small specimens, wet cassette sponges with formalin prior to placement of the tissue in cassettes.

Areas of inflammation are often found adjacent to nasal neoplasms, and multiple biopsies are recommended to ensure representative sampling.

Nasal bacterial and fungal cultures must be interpreted with caution and in light of the histologic and clinical findings. Primary bacterial rhinitis is rare. Most cases of bacterial rhinitis are secondary to other diseases. *Aspergillus* sp. is a common contaminant and diagnosis of fungal rhinitis should not be based on culture results alone. Demonstration of fungal elements in biopsied nasal tissue confirms a diagnosis of fungal rhinitis.

ii   Lung

Indications for pulmonary biopsies include suspected neoplasia or infections of unknown etiology. Bleeding diatheses are contraindications. Biopsy specimens can be collected via thoracotomy, thoracoscopy, or transthoracic needle biopsy. Thoracotomy is the most invasive method, but provides the largest and therefore most representative biopsy specimens. In addition, mass lesions can often be completely removed and the surgery can play a therapeutic role.

While less invasive, thoracoscopy and transthoracic needle biopsies provide relatively small specimens that may not be fully representative of the lesion. The major risks of these procedures are pneumothorax and pulmonary hemorrhage. Other risks include hemothorax, air embolism, hemopericardium, and spread of the tumor. The accuracy of thoracoscopy and pulmonary needle biopsies depends on size and location of the pulmonary nodule, as well as operator expertise.

When available, immediate cytologic evaluation of a smear of the tissue can greatly increase the diagnostic accuracy of the pulmonary needle biopsy by insuring the presence of diagnostic material prior to termination of the biopsy procedure and submission for histopathology.

14   Reproductive

i   Female

Definitive diagnosis of reproductive tract disease often requires biopsy. Indications for female reproductive tract biopsy include pyometra, mass lesions,

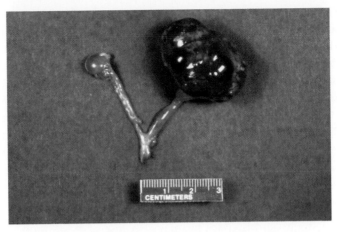

Figure 30 Ovariohysterectomy specimen from a gerbil with a unilateral ovarian tumor (granulosa cell tumor in this case) and a contralateral ovarian cyst.

suspected hermaphroditism, ovarian cystic disease, and infertility. Except in cases of infertility, ovariohysterectomy and submission of the entire tract is often the procedure of choice (Figure 30), as it is both diagnostic, and often curative, but ovarian, uterine (endometrial or full-thickness specimens), or vaginal samples can be submitted. Uterine stumps can be submitted in cases of suspected stump pyometra and ovarian pedicles when residual ovarian tissue is suspected.

While common in rabbits and occasionally seen in guinea pigs and pigs, endometrial carcinoma is exceedingly rare in most other veterinary patients, including cats and dogs. Uterine and vaginal mass lesions in cats and dogs are usually hyperplastic or benign neoplasms and ovariohysterectomy is curative. Ovarian tumors can be benign or malignant.

Equine and canine endometrial biopsies are submitted in cases of infertility and as part of pre-purchase evaluation of potential brood mares. Pregnancy is the only known contraindication (Snider *et al.* 2011). Endometrial biopsies can be collected at any stage of the estrus cycle, but conditions are optimal during estrus when the cervix is relaxed and immune function is high. While it has been reported that, in the horse, a single endometrial biopsy of at least 10 × 3 × 3 mm is fully representative if there are no palpable abnormalities (Kenney & Doig 1986), one study found that 55% of mares had a difference of a grade among three endometrial samples (Dybdal *et al.* 1991).

Gentle handing of endometrial tissue is important to avoid squeeze artifact, loss of superficial epithelium, and herniation of glands.

Bouin's fixative is often recommended for endometrial biopsies because it hardens the tissues and preserves cellular detail well, but formalin-fixed endometrial biopsies are of acceptable quality and avoid the added health and safety concerns associated with the use of Bouin's solution. If Bouin's is used, the tissue should be transferred to 10% formalin or 70% alcohol within 24 hours to prevent overhardening.

Equine endometrial biopsies are graded according to Kenney and Doig's histologic classification of endometrial changes based on degree and extent of inflammatory, fibrotic, lymphatic, and atrophic lesions. The grades are associated with estimations of the mare's ability to bring a foal to term, but must be adjusted according to the number of years the mare has been barren and method of breeding. Supplying the pathologist with the reproductive history, stage of the cycle, and physical findings will help provide accurate grading of the endometrial changes.

ii   Male

Testicles are usually submitted for histology because of mass lesions or for asymmetry. Occasionally the normal testicle is mistaken for the abnormal testicle, and canine primary testicular neoplasms are often multiple and bilateral. Thus, both testicles should be submitted.

Indications for prostatic biopsy include prostatomegaly and dysuria. Prostatic biopsies can be obtained by needle biopsy or open surgical technique. The percutaneous needle method is the least invasive, but is less certain to yield fully representative samples and is contraindicated in cases of cavitary disorders, such as cysts and abscesses. If performing needle biopsies, ultrasound or laparoscopy guidance and multiple samples can increase the likelihood of retrieving diagnostic tissue. When using the open surgery method, care must be taken to avoid damaging the prostatic urethra.

15   Endocrine

i   Thyroid

Thyroids are usually biopsied when neoplasia is suspected. In cats, they are also removed and submitted for histopathology in cases of hyperthyroidism.

While most thyroid tumors are located in the ventral neck, thyroid tissue (and therefore, thyroid tumors) can be found anywhere from the base of the tongue to the base of the heart. Tumors that are fixed in position suggest invasive growth and carcinoma, whereas freely movable tumors are more likely to be benign. Histologic confirmation requires examination of the interface between the tumor and the adjacent tissue for the presence or absence of invasive growth. Thus, needle and incisional biopsies are often of limited use. Additionally, as thyroid tumors are generally highly vascular, needle and incisional biopsies can cause significant and even fatal hemorrhage. Excisional biopsy is recommended.

The majority of cats with hyperthyroidism have bilateral thyroid disease, often requiring bilateral thyroidectomy. Care must be taken to preserve the parathyroid glands.

ii Adrenal gland

Adrenal gland masses can be primary or metastatic. If they are primary, they can be hyperplastic or neoplastic (benign or malignant) and functional (hormone-producing) or non-functional. Clinical findings (including blood pressure), serum biochemical analysis, CBC, imaging studies (size of the adrenal mass and presence or absence of invasive growth and other masses), and endocrine testing can help narrow the differential diagnosis before the decision to biopsy is made. The relevant findings should be provided on the biopsy submission form to help with interpretation of the histologic findings.

Histologic differentiation between benign and malignant primary adrenal gland tumors largely depends on the presence or absence of invasive growth, which cannot be adequately assessed from needle biopsy specimens. In addition, needle biopsies of adrenal gland tumors are associated with risk of hemorrhage, arrhythmias, seeding neoplastic tissue along the needle tract, and so on. While adrenalectomy is associated with a high incidence of perioperative complications, it is diagnostic and can be therapeutic (Schwartz *et al.* 2008).

Adrenocortical disease (unilateral or bilateral hyperplasia, adenoma, and/or carcinoma) is very common in ferrets and is associated with alopecia, vulvar swelling in females, and, sometimes, squamous metaplasia and cyst formation of the prostate in males. Adrenalectomy is the recommended treatment.

iii Parathyroid gland

Parathyroid masses are occasionally encountered. Knowledge of the clinical and surgical findings helps differentiate between chief cell hyperplasia and adenoma of the parathyroid gland. In cases of chief cell hyperplasia, enlargement of at least two parathyroid glands is usually apparent grossly, whereas the vast majority of adenomas involve only a single gland. Parathyroid carcinoma is rare, but histological differentiation between benign chief cell proliferations and adenocarcinoma is largely based on the presence or absence of invasive growth. Therefore, excisional biopsy is recommended.

16 Central nervous system

Clinical signs, imaging studies, serological testing, CSF taps, and electroencephalograms are used to form a differential diagnosis for central nervous system (CNS) lesions, but biopsies are often required to reach a definitive diagnosis, guide treatment, and determine prognosis. Excisional or debulking biopsies can also be used as part of therapy, eliminating or reducing tumor load and allowing for decompression of pre- or post-surgical brain swelling.

Biopsy specimens can be collected via ultrasound-guided or stereotactic-guided needle biopsy, open craniotomy or laminectomy, and require specialized equipment and training. Intraoperative cytology can confirm that lesional tissue was sampled and help determine if material should be submitted for culture. While the difficulty and danger involved in sampling the CNS often results in small and fragmented tissue specimens, it should be remembered that the larger and more intact the specimens, the greater the chance of reaching a definitive and specific diagnosis.

Providing the signalment, relevant clinical history, other test results, and specific location of the tumor, that is, the area of the brain or segment of the spinal cord and the relationship to the dura, parenchyma, and ventricles, will help the pathologist reach an accurate diagnosis.

17 Skeletal muscle

Muscle biopsies are used in cases of neuromuscular disease. While routine light microscopy is sufficient and necessary for the identification of inflammatory myopathies and can identify the specific etiology in some cases, other neuromuscular diseases require fiber typing, enzyme assays, and storage material analysis (not all laboratories perform all of these analyses). Depending on the differential diagnosis based on the clinical signs, blood work results (including creatine kinase [CK] and serology) and electromyography (EMG), formalin-fixed plus or minus fresh, chilled muscle tissue should be submitted. If submitting formalin-fixed muscle tissue and the specimen is not fixed at resting length, the specimens should sit for about 10 minutes before fixation to help minimize the formation of contraction bands (Dubowitz *et al*. 2013) (Figures 31 and 32). If submitting fresh muscle tissue, the specimens can be wrapped in gauze that has been soaked in chilled sterile saline and tightly squeezed out, placed in a hard container, and shipped overnight on ice.

Muscle specimens are best collected via an open surgical approach, but punch biopsies (for superficial muscles) and Bergstrom needle biopsies (for deeper muscles) can be used.

Selection of the muscle to biopsy is based on the muscles affected and the differential diagnosis. Muscles traumatized by EMG studies should be avoided, but those contralateral to muscles that have EMG abnormalities are good candidates. Very weak/atrophied muscles are likely to be end stage and may no longer have diagnostic histologic features. Injections sites should also be avoided. If canine masticatory muscle myositis is suspected, the temporalis and/or masseter muscles should be sampled; lesions in this condition can be patchy and more than one specimen is recommended. When considering equine exertional rhabdomyolysis, including equine polysaccharide storage myopathy, a sample of the semimembranosus muscles is commonly submitted. For diagnosis of equine motor disease, biopsy of the sacrocaudalis dorsalis muscles, which contain more than 20% slow-twitch fibers, is recommended.

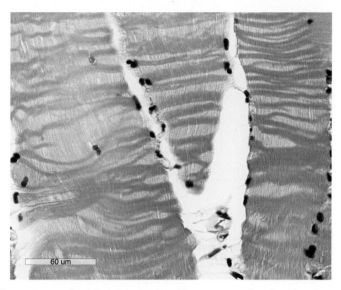

Figure 31 Photomicrograph of skeletal muscle with contraction band artifact distorting the tissue.

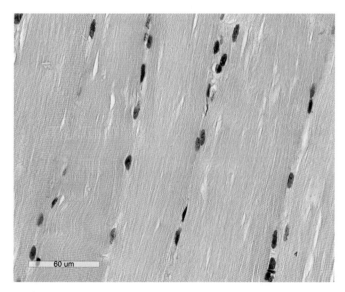

Figure 32 Photomicrograph of the same skeletal muscle depicted in Figure 31 without the contraction band artifact.

18 Miscellaneous

i Anal sacs

Anal sacs are biopsied for mass lesions and in cases of chronic inflammation. The vast majority of anal sac masses are adenocarcinoma of the apocrine glands of the anal sac and excisional biopsy is recommended. Many dogs with adenocarcinoma of the apocrine glands of the anal sac have metastasis to the sublumbar lymph nodes at the time of diagnosis, which is associated with a shorter survival time and disease-free interval (Potanas *et al.* 2015). Therefore, preoperative imaging studies are recommended. Rarely, these tumors are bilateral. Both sacs should be checked.

ii Synovium

Unless a mass lesion is present, synovial biopsies are often not helpful. Synovitis is rarely specific as to cause. Trauma-induced synovitis, infectious synovitis, and autoimmune synovitis can have similar histologic appearances. Number and distribution of joints involved, radiographs, cytology, cultures, and serology can help in reaching a more specific diagnosis.

Biopsy Submission Check List[*]

1. Collection
   a. Appropriate site selection
   b. Appropriate size and number
   c. Appropriate type and amount of fixative; samples are 1 cm or less in thickness
   d. Appropriate labeling – patient, site, orientation, and margins
2. Submission form
   a. Accurate signalment
   b. Pertinent history
   c. Lesion description – number, location, distribution, size, color, shape, consistency
   d. Differential diagnosis and specific questions
3. Clinicopathologic correlation
   a. Review biopsy results in context of clinical history, other lab tests, and response to treatment
   b. Consultation with pathologist regarding any inconsistencies between clinical and histological assessment

[*]Modified from Mouser, P. (2012) Maximizing Biopsy Submissions. *Mass Vet News*, Massachusetts Veterinary Medical Associations, Marlborough, MA, pp. 9–10. Adapted with permission of Dr. Pamela Mouser.

List of Biopsy Dos and Don'ts[*]

DO submit representative and sufficient tissue, including some adjacent normal tissue when possible.

DO fix tissue immediately in sufficient fixative.

DO use a wide-mouth container for fixation.

DO handle the tissue carefully to avoid squeeze artifact.

DO submit signalment and pertinent history and clinical findings.

DON'T incise a small specimen – excise it.

DON'T use electrocautery or lasers on small biopsy specimens.

DON'T put fresh tissue in tissue cassettes with dry cassette sponges.

DON'T freeze biopsy specimens for histopathology.

[*]Modified from Melrose RJ and Handlers JP: Biopsy Dos and Don'ts. http://oralpathology associates.com/Doctors/dosdonts.html. Adapted with permission of Dr. Raymond Melrose.

References

American Veterinary Medical Association. *Required Training for Packaging and Shipping Lab Specimens*, [Online], Available: https://www.avma.org/PracticeManagement/Administration/Pages/Required-Training-for-Packaging-and-Shipping-Lab-Specimens.aspx [14 Sept 2015].

Ashbaugh, E.A. *et al.* (2011) Nasal hydropulsion: a novel tumor biopsy technique *J Amer Anim Hosp Assoc* **47**, 312–316.

Cole, T.L. *et al.* (2002) Diagnostic Comparison of needle and wedge biopsy specimens of the liver in dogs and cats *J Am Vet Med Assoc* **220**, 1483–1490.

Cordner, A.P. *et al.* (2011) Effect of pancreatic tissue sampling on serum pancreatic enzyme levels in clinically heathy dogs *J Vet Diagn Invest* **22**, 702–707.

Cornell, K., & Fischer, J. (2003) Surgery of the exocrine pancreas. In: *Textbook of Small Animal Surgery*, Vol **2**, (ed D Slatter), 3rd edn, p. 754. Saunders, Philadelphia, PA.

Dubowitz, V. *et al.* (2013) Ultrastructural changes. In: *Muscle Biopsy: A Practical Approach*. (ed V. Dubowitz *et al.*), 4th edn, pp. 95. Saunders, China.

Dybdal, N.O. *et al.* (1991) Investigation of the reliability of a single endometrial biopsy sample, with a note on the correlation between uterine cysts on biopsy grade. *J Reprod Fertil* **44**, 697.

Evans, S.E. *et al.* (2006) Comparison of endoscopic and full-thickness biopsy specimens for diagnosis of inflammatory bowel disease and alimentary tract lymphoma in cats. *J Am Vet Med Assoc* **229**, 1447–1450.

Geller, S.A. (1994) Liver biopsy for the nonpathologist. In: *Principles and Practice of Gastroenterology and Hepatology*. (ed G. Gitnick), 2nd edn, pp. 1023–1036. Appleton & Lange, Norwalk, CT.

Golden, D.L. (1993) Gastrointestinal endoscopic biopsy techniques. *Vet Clin North Am Small Anim Pract* **8**, 239.

Harris, B.J. *et al.* (2014) Diagnostic accuracy of three biopsy techniques in 117 dogs with intranasal neoplasia. *J Small Anim Pract* **55**, 219–224.

Kenney, R.M. & Doig, P.A (1986) Equine endometrial biopsy. In: *Current Therapy in Theriogenology* **2**. (ed D.A. Morrow), pp. 723–729. WB Saunders, Philadelphia.

Lees, G.E. *et al.* (2011) Renal biopsy and pathologic evaluation of glomerular disease. *Topics Comp Anim Med* **26**, 143–153.

Melrose, R.J. & Handlers, J.P. *Biopsy Dos and Don'ts*, [Online], Available: http://oralpathology-associates.com/Doctors/dosdonts.html [14 Sept 2015].

Mouser, P. (2012) Maximizing Biopsy Submissions, *Mass Vet News*, Massachusetts Veterinary Medical Associations, Marlborough, MA, pp. 9–10.

Norsworthy G.D. *et al.* (2015) Prevalence and underlying causes of histologic abnormalities in cats suspected to have chronic small bowel disease: 300 cases (2008-2013). *J Am Vet Med Assoc* **247**, 629–635.

Potanas, C.P. *et al.* (2015) Surgical excision of anal sac apocrine gland adenocarcinomas with and without adjunctive chemotherapy in dogs: 42 cases (2005-2011). *J Amer Vet Med Assoc* **246**, 877–884.

Pratschke, K.M. *et al.* (2015) Pancreatic surgical biopsy in 24 dogs and 19 cats: postoperative complications and clinical relevance of histological findings. *J Sm Anim Pract* **56**, 60–66.

Schwartz, P. *et al.* (2008) Evaluation of prognostic factors in the surgical treatment of adrenal gland tumors in dogs: 41 cases (1999-2005). *J Am Vet Med Assoc* **232**, 77–84.

Snider, T.A. *et al.* (2011) Equine endometrial biopsy reviewed: observation, interpretation and application of histopathologic data. *Theriogenology* **75**, 1567–1581.

Sorenmo, K.U. *et al.* (2009) Canine mammary gland tumours; a histological continuum from benign to malignant; clinical and histopathological evidence. *Vet Comp Oncology* **7**, 162–172.

Susaneck, S.J. *et al.* (1983) Inflammatory mammary carcinoma in the dog. *J Amer Anim Hosp Assoc* **19**, 971–976.

U.S. Department of Transportation Pipeline and Hazardous Materials Safety Administration. (2007) *Transporting Infectious Substances Safely*, [Online], Available: http://www.phmsa.dot.gov/pv_obj_cache/pv_obj_id_54AC1BCBF0DFBE298024C4C700569893C2582700/filename/Transporting_Infectious_Substances_brochure.pdf [14 Sept 2015].

Vaden, S.L. (2005) Renal biopsy of dogs and cats. *Clin Tech Sm Anim Pract* **20**, 11–22.

Vaden, S.L. *et al.* (2005) Renal biopsy: a retrospective study of methods and complications in 283 dogs and 65 cats. *J Vet Intern Med* **19**, 794–801.

Willard, M.D. *et al.* (2001) Quality of tissue specimens obtained endoscopically from the duodenum of dogs and cats. *J Amer Vet Med Assoc* **219**, 474–479.

Additional Reading

Aleman, M. (2009) *Muscle biopsy*, [Online], Available: http://www.vetmed.ucdavis.edu/vsr/Neurology/Downloads/Equine%20Muscle%20Biopsy.pdf [14 Sept 2015].

Angus, J.C. (2005) Better skin biopsies, maximize your diagnostic results. *Proceeding of the NAVC*, North American Veterinarian Conference, Orlando, FL, pp. 231–232.

Cianciolo, R.E. *et al.* (2013) Pathologic evaluation of canine renal biopsies: methods for identifying features that differentiate immune-mediated glomerulonephritides from other categories of glomerular disease. *J Vet Intern Med* **27**, S10–S18.

Cullen, J.M. & Van Winkle, T.J. (2007) *Pathology of the liver: what's new and what's still true*. The C.L. Davis Foundation Presentation at the American College of Veterinary Pathologists Annual Meeting, Savannah, GA.

Evans, J. *et al.* (2004) Canine inflammatory myopathies: a clinicopathologic review of 200 cases. *J Vet Intern Med* **18**, 679–691.

Jergens, A.E. & Moore, F.M. (1999) Endoscopic biopsy specimen collection and histopathologic considerations. In: *Small Animal Endoscopy*. (ed T.R. Tams), pp. 323–340. Mosby Year Book Inc, St. Louis.

Kamstock, DA *et al.* (2008) How to and how not to submit your biopsy specimens, [Online], Available: http://csu-cvmbs.colostate.edu/Documents/vdl-biopsy-submission.pdf [14 Sept 2015].

Mauldin, E. (2014) Recommendations for optimizing quality in skin biopsy samples, [Online], Available: http://www.vet.upenn.edu/docs/default-source/ryan/lab-at-ryan-hospital/optimal-skin-biopsy-sampling-guidelines.pdf?sfvrsn=2 [14 Sept 2015].

Moissonnier, P. *et al.* (2002) Stereotactic CT-guided brain biopsy in the dog. *J Sm Anim Pract* **43**, 115–123.

Nowacek, J.M. (2010) Fixation and tissue processing. Revised and updated by JA Kiernan. In: *Special Stains and H&E*. (eds G.L. Kumar & J.A. Kiernan), 2nd edn, pp. 141–143. DAKO, Carpinteria, CA.

Pinson, D.M. (2014) Writing diagnostic laboratory requisition form histories. *J Amer Vet Med Assoc* **244**, 408–411.

Prichard, R.W. (1955) Descriptions in Pathology. *Amer Med Assoc Archives of Pathol* **59**, 612–617.

Rothuizen, J. & Twedt, D.C. (2009) Liver Biopsy Techniques. *Vet Clin Sm Anim* **39**, 469–480.

Sleiman, R. *et al.* (2013) Maximizing diagnostic outcomes of skin biopsy specimens. *International J Derm* **52**, 72–78.

Stromberg, P.C. (2009) *The principles and practice of veterinary surgical pathology*. CL Davis Foundation Workshop. ACVP Annual Meeting. Monterey, CA.

Wilcock, B. (2006) *Common biopsies that may be almost worthless*, [Online], Available: http://www.histovet.com/pdf/HIS_TenWorstBiopsies.pdf [14 Sept 2015].

Wilcock, B. (2006) *Diseases of the canine digit*, [Online], Available: http://www.histovet.com/pdf/HIS_DiseasesCanine.pdf [14 Sept 2015].

Index

Veterinarian's Guide to Maximizing Biopsy Results, First Edition. F. Yvonne Schulman.
© 2016 John Wiley & Sons, Ltd. Published 2016 by John Wiley & Sons, Ltd.